THE MOST PAINFUL BOOK YOU'LL EVER READ

DR. STEVEN LOCKSTONE
Chiropractor | B.App.Sc.(Clin.Sc.)/B.C.Sc. RMIT

Copyright © 2021 Dr Steven Lockstone B.App.Sc.(Clin.Sc.)/B.C.Sc. RMIT Chiropractor | Wellness Influencer | Speaker

ISBN-

ALL RIGHTS RESERVED

No part of this book may be reproduced or transmitted in any form whatsoever, electronic, or mechanical, including photocopying, recording, or by any informational storage or retrieval without the publisher's expressed written consent, except in the brief quotation in critical articles or reviews.

The author and publisher have provided this book to you for your personal use only. You may not make this book publicly available in any way. Criminal copyright infringement, including infringement without monetary gain, is punishable by law. If you believe the copy of this book, you are reading infringes on the author's copyright, please notify the publisher.

First Edition

Printed in Australia.

LEGAL NOTICES
The information contained in this book, including but not limited to text, graphics, images and other material, is for educational purposes only. It is based upon the research and personal and professional experience of the author. It is not intended as a substitute for professional medical advice, diagnosis or treatment. Any attempt to diagnose and treat an illness should be done under the direction of a healthcare professional.

Regardless of your current state of health, always seek the advice of your physician or other qualified health care provider with any questions you may have regarding your current health condition, a medical condition or treatment, and before undertaking a new health care regimen. Never disregard professional medical advice or delay in seeking it because of something you have read in this book.

The publisher and author do not advocate the use of any particular healthcare protocol but believes the information in this book should be available to the public. The publisher and author are not responsible for any adverse effects or consequences resulting from the use of the suggestions, procedures, products and services discussed in this book. Should the reader have any questions concerning the appropriateness of any procedures or products mentioned, the author and publisher strongly suggest consulting with a professional healthcare adviser.

Results May Vary
The information presented herein represents the view of the author as of the date of publication. Because of the rate with which conditions change, the author reserve the right to alter and update his opinion based on the new conditions. This book is for informational purposes only. While every attempt has been made to verify the information provided in this book, neither the authors nor their affiliates/partners assume any responsibility for errors, inaccuracies or omissions. Any slights of people or organisations are unintentional.

TERMS AND CONDITIONS OF USE AND COPYRIGHT NOTICE
Please be advised that this program is for informational purposes only and is based on the clinical experiences of the doctor / author.

DISCLAIMER
This book is a book for the layperson and is not intended to be a professional manual. It is designed to provide information about the subject matter covered. It is sold with the understanding that the publisher and author are not engaged in rendering medical advice. The information in this book is non-diagnostic and is not intended to replace medical treatment. If medical or other expert assistance is required, a licensed healthcare professional's services should be sought. The purpose of this book is to educate and entertain.

The publisher, author, or any dealer or distributor shall not be liable to the purchaser or any other person or entity with respect to any liability, loss, or damage caused or alleged to be caused directly or indirectly by this book.

Dedication

To my parents, Netty and Rusty, who kept pushing me when times got tough and supported me so that I could focus on becoming a chiropractor. (ps. I won't forget the 4 am wake up calls during exam time lol)

To the thousands of people who have trusted me with their health over the past 20 years and who chose to not be dependent on drugs or surgery but rather acknowledge that the power that made the body heals the body and if the body is healing and functioning the way it was intended to, then we can live a life of abundant, vibrant health.

To all the Chiropractors that have come before me, thank you!

Acknowledgments

Thanks to Dr Abe Kaplan DC for fixing my back and inspiring me to become a chiropractor.

Thanks to Dr David Cohen DC for encouraging me to become a chiropractor.

Thanks to Professor Kleynhans, who helped me transition from Chiropractic University in South Africa to Australia at a moment's notice.

Thanks to Dr David Hendrey (Chiro) for introducing me to "wellness" Chiropractic and for the countless hours spent observing him in practice, helping with spinal screenings and attending seminars.

Thanks to Dr Jens Sorensen (Chiro), for taking me to my first chiropractic philosophy night.

Thanks to Dr Stephen Franson DC for his guidance around the 10 questions used as the theme in this book and for his continued mentorship.

Thanks to Dr Bobby Ilijasevic (Chiro) for coaching me on how to have a remarkable practice as part of a remarkable life.

Thanks to Adrian Falk for coming up with the title for this book.

Thanks to my gorgeous wife, Martine, for encouraging me to write this book and share my story so that others may benefit from this healing art.

Finally, a humble thanks to the Universe for blessing me with an abundance of health, happiness and the joy I receive every day in using my gift of healing others.

Contents

My Back Story.. 1
Is This Book About You? 7
Are You Designed to be Healthy or Sick? 14
Is Your Body Smart or Stupid?.................................... 20
Which is the Most Important System in
    Your Body for Staying Healthy?...................... 23
What Protects Your Nervous System? 27
Is Your Life Stressful?... 31
What Does Chronic Stress Do to Your Body? 37
What is the Root Cause of Most
    Health Problems? 43
How is Your Nervous System Functioning? 51
How to Correct Problems with
    Your Nervous System? 55
When is the Best Time to Take Care of
    Your Health? 60
Universal Truths 62
Fibs, Tales and Lies 66
A New Beginning 74
References 76

List of Tables, Figures and Diagrams

Table
Table 1: Pre-existing comorbidities in patients with COVID-19

Figures
Figure 1: Chronic disorders in patients with COVID-19
Figure 2: Main comorbidities among COVID-19 deaths in New York

Diagrams
Diagram 1: the nervous system
Diagram 2: the subluxation complex
Diagram 3: text neck
Diagram 4: body imbalance
Diagram 5: the Safety Pin Cycle

My Back Story

I believe that the greatest gift you can give your family and the world is a healthy you.
~Joyce Meyer

If you have ever heard me speak at one of my public talks on chiropractic, you would be forgiven for thinking that I was fresh off the boat from South Africa. Truth be told, I immigrated to Australia from Johannesburg, South Africa, to continue my chiropractic studies in 1996. Yet my South African accent is as strong as the day I left.

I come from a warm and loving family. My mum, Annette, was a hairdresser and my dad, Russel, owned a hardware store. I have a younger brother, Ryan.

I was also privileged to grow up close to my grandparents. When my grandmother, "Boobii", died, my grandfather, Abe, moved in permanently and even immigrated with us to Australia.

I have a funny memory of studying chiropractic: I knew how many hours of study I had done each day by the number of empty cups of tea on my desk because I had asked my grandfather to bring me a fresh cup every hour.

I have fond memories of growing up in South Africa. It's a beautiful place and full of cultural flavour, stunning landscapes and a pulse that, let's say, keeps you on your toes!

I moved to Sydney in 2014 and met my beautiful wife, Martine, just two weeks in. We got married in 2017 and have been blessed with two beautiful children, Allie and Axel, oh and don't forget the cats, Pyke and Bella.

Back to my early years ...

As a kid, I did not grow. At the age of 17, I had the body of a 12-year-old. I was being bullied by my fellow students, and it was clear to my mother that there was something wrong.

Our family GP suggested a therapy that he was using with other kids. It involved giving hormone injections that caused the body to release human growth hormone (HGH) and therefore stimulated the growth of every cell in the body, including those cells that turn a boy into a man. After just three treatments, I began to grow rapidly.

Due to the rapid growth, my body could not lay down enough calcium into the bones, which resulted in the vertebrae developing a wedge-like shape. The result was a condition known as Scheuermann's disease. I recall the doctor telling my mother that I had this "disease", and as you could imagine, it shocked her. But it's more of a condition than a disease.

As a result of Scheuermann's Disease, I developed raging sciatica and will never forget the excruciating and agonising sharp stabbing and hot poker pain in my legs that had me on the floor crying for help.

After trying numerous physiotherapists and massage therapists, I was referred to Dr Abe Kaplan, a chiropractor. After a few treatments, my sciatica resolved, and it became a distant memory.

After school, I travelled around Europe and Israel for about 18 months with a couple of good friends, Dino and Idan. We were having an amazing time until I got that fateful call from my mum.

"What do you want to do with your life?" she asked. Well, I had things planned out. I was going back to the kibbutz to work in the fridges during the hot desert summer. However, my mum clarified that working in a fridge in the desert was not an appropriate career choice and that I had been accepted for an interview with the Chiropractic School in Johannesburg.

To cut a long story short, two weeks later, I was enrolled into the University of Witwatersrand and sitting in the first of many anatomy classes.

On the morning after my 21st Birthday Party, my cousin Justin woke me up with the news that my mother had been hijacked at gun point in the driveway to our home, but thankfully she managed to get away and survived. That incident rattled the whole family, and we took decisive action.

I called the Head of the Chiropractic School in Melbourne, who I had stopped in to say hello on a recent trip to Melbourne. I asked if he could make a place for me at RMIT Chiropractic, to which he replied, *"a Boer Maak a Plan"*, meaning "A Farmer Makes a Plan".

Three months later, I left for Australia in February 1996 as an international student, while my family settled their affairs and the entire family prepared to immigrate.

As the course was structured differently from my WITS Chiropractic course, I had to start again, although I did have course credits scattered through the RMIT course. Nonetheless, another five years of study began.

I delved deep into the philosophy of chiropractic by attending group philosophy nights hosted by various students frequently, often volunteering my body to the senior students so they could practice their adjustments and teach me how to adjust! I loved every minute of the course and the culture that surrounded me.

In my third year, I had a fateful introduction to a local chiropractor, a wellness chiropractor. At his practice, my eyes were opened to the real application of chiropractic wellness principles. His practice was "open plan", with two tables side by side. The atmosphere was vibrant, holistic and positive. People were practice members, not patients. The chiropractor was giving out high fives and hugs, and everyone was happy.

I was hooked! I did everything I could to be close to the chiropractor, processing his X-rays, cleaning the whiteboards, changing the paper towel for patients—anything I could do to help and just absorb the atmosphere he had created.

One of the key ingredients that I learned from him was to go out to the public and educate through "spinal screenings", where you check peoples' posture and educate them on the benefits of spinal health.

I started doing screenings for him and also began doing screenings for many other chiropractors. Over the years, I introduced over 12,000 people to various chiropractors across Victoria.

During my fourth year of chiropractic school, I decided to open my own chiropractic clinic and employ some chiropractors to do the work. I was the first and only student to have done this, and it created quite a stir among the profession. By the time I graduated, I had three chiropractors working for me and opened my second practice immediately after graduating.

I've written this book for you so that you can understand how chiropractic care may optimise your health and enhance your quality of life.

Dr Steven Lockstone
B.App.Sc.(Clin.Sc.)/B.C.Sc. RMIT
Chiropractor | Wellness Influencer | Speaker

Connect with me: mychiro.com.au/DrSteve

Is This Book About You?

A healthy outside starts from the inside.
~Robert Urich

Imagine for a moment that this was a book about your life and health choices.

Over the last few years, you have had to repeatedly deal with back pain, neck pain, headaches, bad posture, or sciatica. You visit your GP, who happily prescribes progressively stronger pills for you to take. Or maybe you go to see the physiotherapist or chiropractor or get a massage once or twice. Or you buy one of those new devices advertised all over Facebook … but you just keep going in circles.

You find yourself making "reactive" lifestyle choices because life is so busy and stressful that you need a quick solution so that you can keep grinding away.

You take painkillers to dull that headache you get from not drinking enough water or staring at the monitor for eight hours or more every day.

You really want to keep looking your best and fit into your favourite denims, so you take anti-inflammatories to keep up your exercise regime.

You think to yourself, "If it doesn't hurt, it can't be that bad, so I'll keep pushing".

You know your diet is not that great. But you don't have time to eat wholesome organic meals that you make at home from fresh ingredients, so you opt for the tasty takeaway meals that are so conveniently delivered to your door.

You know that you need to drink more water but let's be realistic, a can of Coke or cup of instant coffee is basically made of water... right?

Your back hurts to get out of bed in the morning, and you need an extra 10 minutes in the shower, with hot water on your back—just so it feels less painful.

You often feel run down or burned out. And if you get a cold, cough, sore throat or fever, you quickly reach for the throat lozenges, antihistamines, paracetamol or sleeping pills because they work so well if you keep taking them.

You notice that your clothes are getting tighter every year, so you try to diet and cut out sugar, carbs and alcohol. But then you realise that they are everywhere and it's more stressful and more expensive to avoid them. So, you just slip back into your old bad habits.

You've seen your older relatives suffer through hip operations, spinal fusions and discectomies to help them manage chronic pain after they realised they just couldn't keep taking those painkillers because they were getting ulcers from the pills.

You've seen your blood pressure slowly rising. You've been told that you are "pre-diabetic" and need to lose weight. Your cholesterol is climbing steadily, and that feeling of anxiety keeps sneaking in. And let's not mention depression ... (You can take a pill for that too!)

You spend hours sitting, staring at your monitor. Your neck has been tight and sore for ages. You can even feel things grating inside. Your hip flexors are so tight that you are starting to slump forward. The hump on your lower neck is becoming more noticeable.

Looking down at your mobile phone affects your sleep. Your insomnia seems to worsen because you are sitting up in bed catching up on emails or social media.

You think you are relatively healthy because health is the opposite of being sick. And you're definitely not sick, at least compared to those visibly sick people who can't live their lives to their full extent. You're not that sick!

You have heard the term "health care", but it sounds like something you'd need if you were sick... and the "sick care model" doesn't seem to fit with you.

Now you have a choice: do you put this book down, or do you turn the page and read on?

Remember, your health is your decision.

Good choice!

So, let's get back to why you think you're not sick!

You've been led to believe that "sick care" is damage control. The obvious need for "sick care" is in emergencies, such as accidents, fractures and other life-or-death acute conditions. Management of chronic conditions like diabetes, heart disease and cancer would also fall into this category.

Here's the ugly truth: the primary goal of "sick care" is just to stop you from getting worse. The secondary goal is to relieve your symptoms and make you feel better. The "sick care" model does not focus on correcting the root cause of your problem. It usually does not move you towards health and prevent the problem from occurring again.

The other side of the coin is "health care", or wellness. You're healthy, right! If you need to run up those stairs, you can, and you can keep getting up every day and going to work. You understand that "wellness" is anything and everything that helps move you towards health and away from illness. Wellness includes nutrition, exercise, wholefood supplements, dental care, chiropractic care, massage and acupuncture.

Think of it this way. You've got some life experience, and you know that life is full of grey areas. It's not simply black and white. So why should it come down to a choice between **sick** or **healthy**?

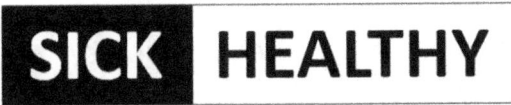

So, if it's not simply black (**SICK**) or white (**HEALTHY**), then there has to be some grey area.

Let's call the grey area **NOT SICK**.

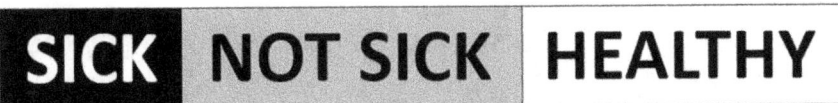

Now that makes more sense.

SICK is where you need medical intervention, drugs or surgery that literally prevent you from getting so sick that you die.

However, **NOT SICK** (the grey area) is quite a broad spectrum that you can move back and forth across:

- You get the flu; you're closer to **SICK**.
- You feel good; you're closer to **HEALTHY**.

You get sicker, or you get healthier, but how do you **stay healthy**?

Well, that depends on where the focus is because we all know that we get what we focus on!

Three broad reasons determine why you are in your current level of health.

First, your health is your responsibility.

Second, you have been given the wrong definition of health until now, so it is not really your fault.

Last, it's procrastination that leads to decay in health, just like everything in life.

If it's left alone, it will decay.

- If you don't brush your teeth, you will get tooth decay.
- If you don't exercise, your muscles will decay (waste away).
- If you don't have healthy habits, your health will decay.

In this book, I'm going to pose 10 simple questions that, if answered honestly, will open the gateway to a life of abundant health and wellness!

1. Are you designed to be healthy or sick?
2. Is your body smart or stupid?
3. What is the most important system your body uses to stay healthy?
4. What protects your nervous system?
5. Is your life stressful?
6. What does stress do to your body?
7. What is the root cause of most health problems?
8. How is YOUR nervous system functioning?
9. What should you do to correct problems with your nervous system?
10. When is the best time to deal with your health?

Let's get started with the first question: Are you designed to be healthy or sick?

Are You Designed to be Healthy or Sick?

Health is a state of complete mental, social and physical wellbeing and not merely the absence of disease or infirmity.
~World Health Organization[1]

Is healthy normal? Is it acceptable in today's society to be "healthy"? I would argue that it is normal to want to be healthy. Who doesn't want good health? Who doesn't want to avoid disease and suffering? Everybody wants to feel young and vibrant, right? But is it the norm? Is being healthy something that people can expect?

According to government stats, the answer is no! Australian Government stats show that in 2019, there were 43,477 deaths due to cardiovascular disease,[2]

---

[1] "Constitution," World Health Organization (WHO), https://www.who.int/about/who-we-are/constitution.
[2] "Heart Disease Statistics," The Heart Foundation, https://www.heartfoundation.org.au/about-us/what-we-do/heart-disease-in-australia/cardiovascular-disease-fact-sheet.

25,116 deaths due to cancer[3] and 1,621 deaths due to prescription drugs.[4]

Let's put that into perspective. Imagine a 747 aeroplane that carries about 450 people. Now imagine that aeroplane falling out of the sky and crashing 156 times a year. That's three times a week, every week with 450 people on board. That's equivalent to 70,000 people dying for only the top three causes of death in Australia. So, what are the chances of anyone being willing to jump on the next flight? Well, the crazy thing is that we do it every day with the lifestyles we accept and the model of health that we follow.

This current health care model is failing

Just think of these common diseases and decide if they are becoming more or less prevalent:

1. obesity
2. diabetes
3. stroke
4. hypertension
5. heart disease
6. ADHD

---

[3] "Deaths in Australia," Australian Institute of Health and Welfare, last modified 7 August 2020, https://www.aihw.gov.au/reports/life-expectancy-death/deaths/data.

[4] "Accidental drug overdose deaths up almost 40 per cent in a decade," Australian Institute of Health and Welfare, last modified 27 August 2019, https://www.abc.net.au/news/health/2019-08-27/accidental-drug-overdoses-forecast-to-reach-record-high/11450764.

7. cancer
8. allergy
9. asthma
10. arthritis
11. infertility
12. depression
13. autoimmune diseases

They are all on the rise, and that's why our current healthcare model is failing. Now think about the COVID-19 global pandemic and how it has stressed health systems around the world. People with chronic disorders such as hypertension or diabetes mellitus are more likely to develop a more severe course of COVID-19. In addition, older patients, especially 65 years old and above with comorbidities, are more likely to die from COVID-19.[5]

Table 1: Pre-existing comorbidities in patients with COVID-19[6]

Comorbidities	Number	Percentage
Hypertension	272	15.8%
Cardiovascular and Cerebrovascular diseases	200	11.7%
Endocrine system (diabetes)	161	9.4%

---

[5] A Sanyaolu et al., "Comorbidity and its Impact on Patients with COVID-19," *SN Comprehensive Clinical Medicine* (2020):1–8, Advance online publication, https://doi.org/10.1007/s42399-020-00363-4.

[6] SS Paudel, "A Meta-Analysis of 2019 Novel Coronavirus Patient Clinical Characteristics and Comorbidities, *Research Square* (2020), http://doi.org/10.21203/rs.3.rs-21831/v1.

Co-existing infection (HIV and Hepatitis B)	25	1.5%
Cancer	25	1.5%
Respiratory (COPD etc.)	24	1.4%
Kidney disorders	14	0.8%
Immunodeficiency states	2	0.01%

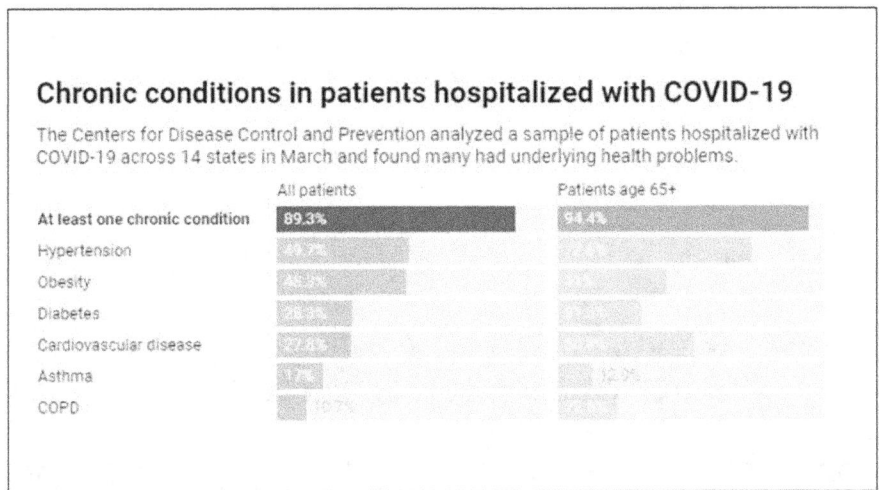

Figure 1: Chronic disorders in patients with COVID-19[7]

---

[7] S Garg et al., "Hospitalization Rates and Characteristics of Patients Hospitalized with Laboratory-Confirmed Coronavirus Disease 2019 — COVID-NET, 14 States, March 1–30, 2020," *MMWR Morbidity & Mortality Weekly Report* 69 (2020): 458–464, http://dx.doi.org/10.15585/mmwr.mm6915e3.

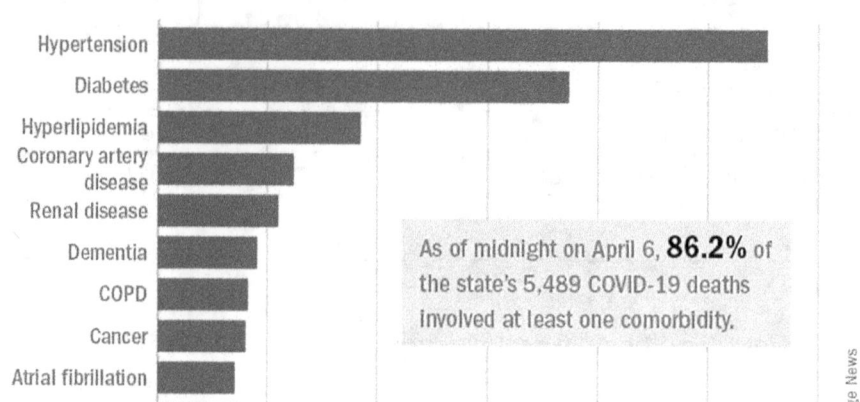

Figure 2: Main comorbidities among COVID-19 deaths in New York[8]

Now consider the top 3–4 conditions: hypertension, diabetes, obesity and hyperlipidaemia. It's not random that these conditions are the most common. They point towards **metabolic syndrome**, which is a cluster of conditions that occur together and include:

- increased blood pressure
- high blood sugar
- excess body fat around the waist
- abnormal cholesterol and/or triglyceride levels.

---

[8] R Franki, "Comorbidities the rule in New York's COVID-19 deaths," *The Hospitalist* (2020), accessed 1 June 2020, https://www.the-hospitalist.org/hospitalist/article/220457/coronavirus-updates/comorbidities-rule-new-yorks-covid-19-deaths].

If you have metabolic syndrome, it increases your risk of heart disease, stroke, and type 2 diabetes[9] and now COVID-19.

So, are we masking the problem by simply taking medications and dealing with the symptoms that these bad lifestyle choices have presented?

It's important to shift the focus away from symptom management (or, in the case of COVID, the strength of the virus) to a wellness approach where we focus on the strength of the host and make our bodies strong and resilient so that we can continue to adapt to the stresses around us.

Healthy is normal—unhealthy is abnormal

You are designed to be healthy. Your body has so much amazing potential. It has the unique ability to heal itself and to function optimally as long as your nervous system is operating without any interference. All you have to do is to unleash its ability to heal itself and live an optimal life.

Healthy is your default. Healthy is normal. The 2000 healthy generations that came before you prove it. Unfortunately, unhealthy is the norm today.

And this leads us to the second question: Is your body smart or stupid?

---

[9] "Metabolic Syndrome," Mayo Clinic, https://www.mayoclinic.org/diseases-conditions/metabolic-syndrome/symptoms-causes/syc-20351916

Is Your Body Smart or Stupid?

Wholeness or health is our natural state. The nature of healing involves removing obstructions to this natural state and bringing individuals into alignment with themselves and their world.
~Richard Carlson

Every living organism has an innate intelligence. Innate intelligence is the intelligence that governs every single act in your body. Every single chemical reaction, the formation of every tissue and the resistance to every invasion are controlled and coordinated by this innate intelligence.

Innate intelligence causes a tree to grow out of a seed. It also causes animals and birds to develop from a single-celled organism. Innate intelligence causes each one of those plants and animals to be what they become.

Your innate intelligence includes your DNA. It transformed you from a one-celled organism into a being with highly complex organs, muscles and bone structures. It knew what to do and which types of cells to create. It knew how to form your heart, liver, kidneys and other organs.

Your innate intelligence directed all these developments, and it continues to direct them even today. It continues to heal you and constantly redevelop your body.

You are a completely new person with completely new cells every 10 years or so. Your organs renew themselves every six weeks; your taste buds renew themselves every ten days; and your entire skeletal structure renews itself every 10 years—all of which is guided by your innate intelligence.

How does it do all this?

- How does your innate intelligence communicate with all of your body parts?
- How does it know how to heal your right thumb when you smash it with a hammer, and at the same time, know how to heal a bacterial infection from a cut in your left foot?
- How does your innate intelligence know how to absorb some nutrients and reject others, and at the same time, know how to grow the muscles that you worked out at the gym?

This innate intelligence is intended to keep us healthy throughout our lifetime.

So, let's not forget how smart our bodies are! Health comes from the inside-out, not the outside-in. And so do sickness and symptoms.

How can you choose to be healthy instead of sick? To figure that out, we have to answer this question: Which is the most important system in your body for staying healthy?

Which is the Most Important System in Your Body for Staying Healthy?

Look to the nervous system as the key to maximum health.
~Galen

The nervous system is the most important in the body because your innate intelligence is transmitted through it. Your innate intelligence controls all the functions and all of your body's organs by communicating through the nervous system via minute electrical impulses.

The nervous system is the communication system that helps us adapt to and deal with stress. The flow of intelligence or information through the nerves keeps us healthy. All our organs depend on the nervous system for optimal health and function. The nervous system also helps us to adapt and deal with stress.

Innate intelligence is present in every cell of your body. However, its command centre is in your brain and spinal cord. The communication network for your innate intelligence is your nervous system. The central nervous system (CNS), which consists of the brain and the spinal cord, sends and receives signals from the Peripheral Nervous System, that is, the nerves in the body.

That information pathway travels from the brain to the spinal cord, then from a small space between two vertebrae in the form of a nerve, which takes the signal to the organs and tissues. If this network is disturbed along this path, the signal will be distorted or even lost.

It is crucial for our body parts to always remain plugged into the innate intelligence network so they can be properly governed while performing their specific tasks and re-forming and healing from injuries. A body part that loses communication with this network stops functioning properly and loses its coordination with the rest of the body. As a result, it becomes weak and vulnerable to breakdown because it can't function or heal properly.

Chiropractic optimises the flow of innate intelligence from your brain to the different parts of the body and thus helps to recover and restore function and start the healing process. The main function of chiropractic is to support your innate intelligence.

Sure, chiropractors help many people relieve their neck and back pain, but that is a by-product of realigning the vertebrae, which restores the innate intelligence network. When a vertebra shifts out of alignment, it not only puts pressure on the nerve, but it also triggers a degenerating process in that joint. The disc will begin to grow weaker, and the joint surfaces will begin to break down and develop arthritis. This will lead to inflammation in that area, increased muscle tension and joint pain.

All of these conditions are also managed through chiropractic care. Most importantly, however, chiropractic allows your innate intelligence to communicate freely throughout the body through your nervous system. As a result, your innate intelligence is programmed to cause your body to thrive when healthy, and it will strive to do so—as long as it has the right tools and is not interfered with.

The nervous system is the most important in the body, so it is vital that it is well-protected.

In the next chapter, we shall see how the body protects your nervous system and keeps it safe and secure.

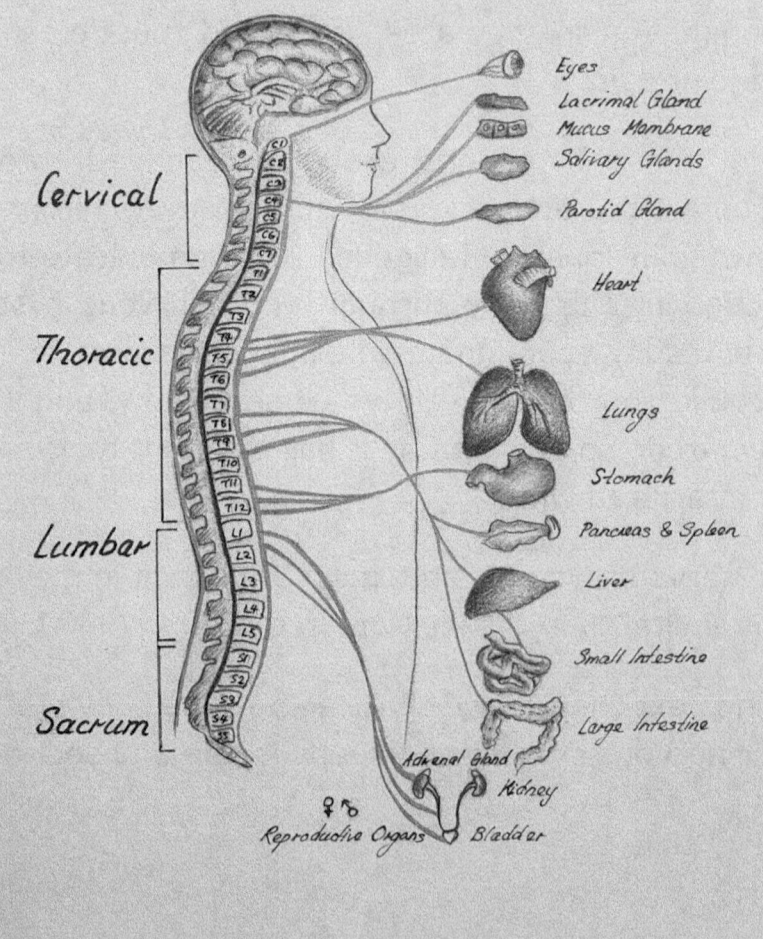

Diagram 1: the nervous system

What Protects Your Nervous System?

If you would seek health, look first to the spine.
~Socrates

If you want to be healthy, you must have a healthy nervous system. And if you want a healthy nervous system, then you must have a healthy spine. Full stop.

Your spine protects your spinal cord, just as your skull protects your brain. The skull is the helmet that protects your brain. Your spine is the suit of armour that protects your spinal cord. Remember, your brain and spinal cord are one continuous system.

The spine protects the spinal cord and the nerve roots that exit from it. These nerves then travel throughout your body, connecting every cell, tissue, joint, muscle and organ, and they regulate their functioning. As long as the nervous system functions well, the body also functions well and recovers quickly from any injury.

The vertebral column's 24 moving bones (vertebrae) play an important role in supporting and protecting the spinal cord and its nerve roots. A loss of the normal motion of these vertebrae due to injury or unhealthy habits can affect the function of the nervous system. Chiropractors refer to this loss of normal motion of the spine as a **subluxation** or **biomechanical joint dysfunction**.

This irritation can affect the neurology and nerve roots exiting the spine and disrupt the transmission of the continuous (electrical) nerve impulses to and from the brain, just like the dimmer switch on a light. Subluxation may result in the weakened performance of the organs or body parts supplied by those nerves. So those organs or muscles may not function properly, and your health will be adversely affected.

Spinal problems often develop gradually and insidiously, similar to tooth decay, heart disease and arthritis. But the "problem" might not be what you think. For example, if someone you know had a heart attack on a Tuesday, were they considered healthy on the Monday?

Spinal joints can get stuck and begin to lose their normal range of motion, leading to the surrounding muscles tightening and localised swelling to avoid further damage.

This abnormal joint movement along with tight muscles and swelling can compress the spinal nerve roots as they exit in between the vertebrae. This interferes with the communication that travels along those nerves between the body and the brain and, in turn, leads to nerve damage and dysfunction.

The process of developing a Vertebral Subluxation complex is subtle. Physical, chemical or emotional stress cause a vertebra to move into an altered state of restricted motion in response to that stress.

A healthy nervous system is essential for health, and a healthy spine is essential for a healthy nervous system. So, you must look after and protect your spine, your suit of armour.

What is the biggest threat to your spine and the leading cause of subluxation? The answer is stress.

How do we protect the spine from all kinds of stress and prevent or minimise subluxations? We shall learn that in the next chapter.

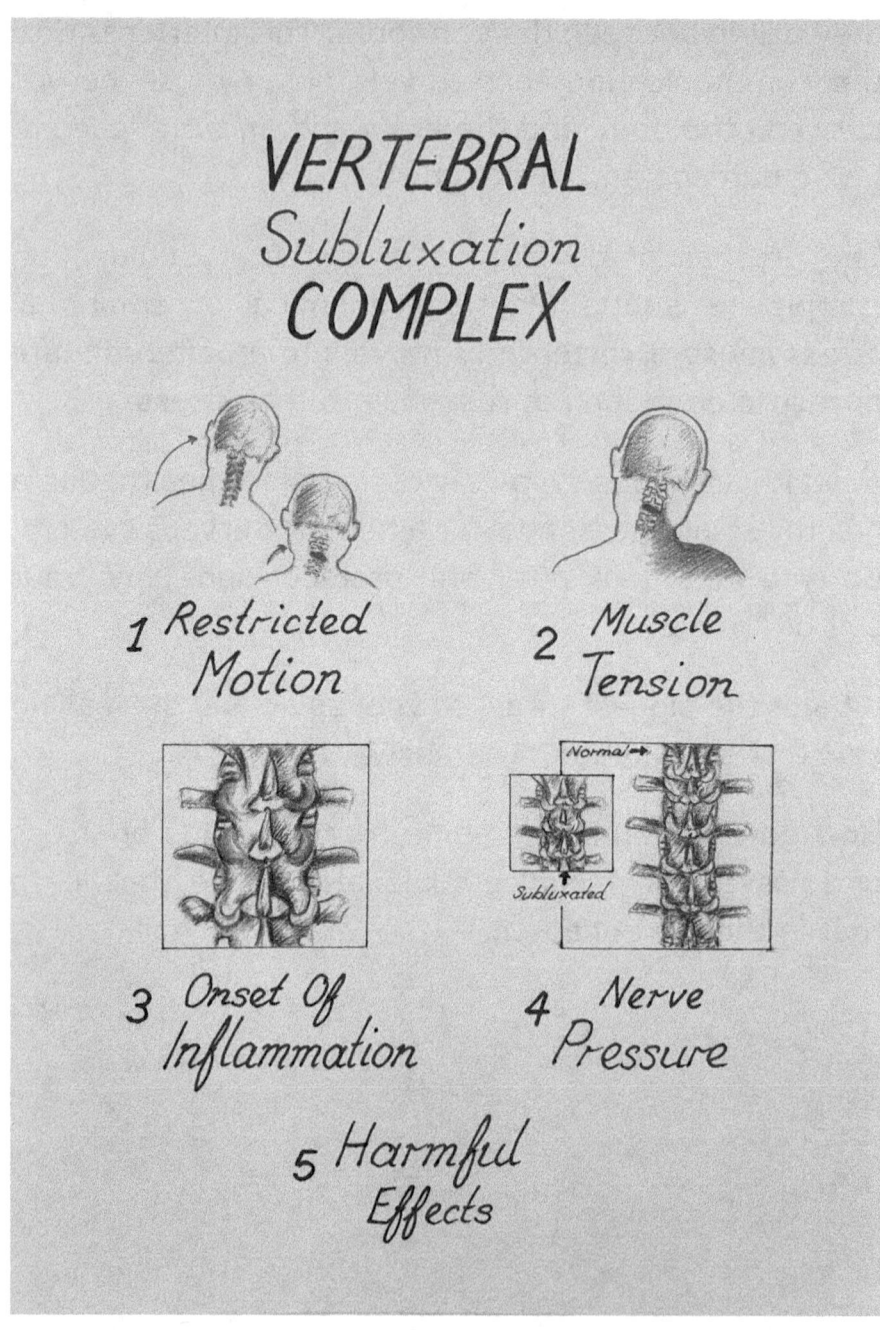

Diagram 2: the subluxation complex

Is Your Life Stressful?

It's not the load that breaks you down; it's the way you carry it.
~Lou Holtz

Stress and strain are how your body and brain respond to any challenge, such as pressures at work or home, financial worries and injuries. Stress is caused by minor and major stressors, which can affect your health and wellbeing. However, some people can handle stress more effectively and recover more quickly than others.

Five important facts about stress

1. Stress affects everyone
2. Not all stress is bad
3. Long-term (chronic) stress can harm your health
4. Ways to manage stress include regular exercise, relaxation activities, sufficient sleep and social support from family and friends
5. If you're overwhelmed by stress, ask for help from a health professional, especially if you feel

overwhelmed, have suicidal thoughts or are using alcohol or drugs to cope with stress[10]

Three types of stress that can contribute to subluxations

The causes of subluxation are **trauma, toxins** and **stress**, which is to say: physical, chemical and emotional stress.

1. **Trauma:** Macro-trauma includes road accidents, sporting injuries, falls, etc., and micro-trauma includes unhealthy lifestyle habits—like looking down at your mobile phone or laptop, poor posture habits such as slouching, wearing high heels, carrying a thick wallet in your back pocket, a lumpy bed, repetitive motion injuries, etc.
2. **Toxins**: These include household chemicals, air pollution, smoke exposure, chemicals in our food such as preservatives and flavouring agents, GMOs, inflammatory foods like sugar and trans fats, chemicals in our water, prescription medications including antibiotics, chemicals that leach from plastic, etc.
3. **Thoughts**: emotional stress can include survival in the rat race, traffic, disharmony at home or work, long working days, financial stress, social anxiety, etc.

---

[10] National Institute of Mental Health. 5 Things You Should Know About Stress. https://www.nimh.nih.gov/health/publications/stress/index.shtml

Stress affects most of us, and we end up feeling overwhelmed because of the pressures we face every single day.

Five common causes of stress

It seems that stress is an inseparable part of modern life. So, let's identify the most common causes so that we can guard against them.

1. Pollution
As already mentioned, we are exposed to increasing levels of air pollution, water pollution, food pollution, household pollution and noise pollution. There is no respite anywhere, and it's only getting worse. All of these forms of pollution affect not only our physical health but also our mental and emotional health.

2. Not doing "first things first"
In the words of Goethe, "Things which matter most must never be at the mercy of things which matter least." Unfortunately, most of us fail to plan and prioritise. So, we feel pulled in 10 different directions at the same time, leading to weariness and frustration at the end of the day.

3. Constantly on the go
Thanks to modern technology, we are connected with our family, friends, colleagues, clients and even absolute strangers throughout the world through our smartphones and computers. Email, Facebook,

LinkedIn, Instagram, WhatsApp, YouTube—it's like being on a lifelong roller coaster ride fuelled by SOS (shiny object syndrome) and FOMO (fear of missing out).[11]

When is the last time you took a digital detox from all your devices for at least a day—or even for a few hours? Perhaps more disturbingly, when is the last time you switched off your smartphone?

4. Trying to be everything to everyone all the time

It isn't possible to be perfect in the office and at home and to excel in every area of life all at the same time. The pressure to be constantly perfect will eventually take its toll. The ultimate and inevitable result is exhaustion and burnout.

5. Poor stress management

Stress is inevitable, but it need not lead to strain and subluxation. Unfortunately, most of us handle stress in the wrong way. Our relieving stress methods are either too **infrequent** (going for a stroll once a week, booking a relaxing massage once a month, etc.) or **counterproductive** (using sugary or fatty comfort foods, caffeine, tobacco, alcohol, drugs, etc.)[12]

---

[11] H Alford, "The Tyranny of Constant Contact," *New York Times*, 17 May 2015, https://www.nytimes.com/2015/05/17/style/the-tyranny-of-constant-contact.html.

[12] "5 reasons why modern life causes stress (and what to do about it)," The Skill Collective, last updated 29 May 2017, https://theskillcollective.com/blog/modern-life-causes-stress.

The human stress response

The amygdala is the part of our brain that detects stress caused by all kinds of stressors. However, the amygdala does not distinguish the type of stressor: real, imagined, mental, emotional, physical, internal or external. Instead, it simply recognises all of them as stress.

We then react instinctively because that's how we are programmed to react. So, we react in the same way to a tight deadline as we would to a crocodile.

The stress response kicks off a chain reaction that includes a range of physiological changes:

- Increased heart rate, respiratory rate and blood pressure
- Anxiety, overwhelm, depression and despair
- Reduced ability to concentrate
- Increased sensitivity to pain
- Increased hormones like cortisol and catecholamines
- Increased glucose and cholesterol levels
- Increased clotting factors
- Decreased anabolic hormones like testosterone and growth hormone
- Decreased immunity
- Insulin resistance
- Bone loss and changes in muscle fibre type.[13]

---

[13] "The Stress Series: Part 1 – Stress Physiology – A Central Theme in Chiropractic?", Australian Spinal Research Foundation, last updated 11 September 2018, https://spinalresearch.com.au/the-stress-series-part-1-stress-physiology-a-central-theme-in-chiropractic/.

To combat stress successfully, we need to take care of our basic building blocks of health.

Next, let us examine the harmful effects of chronic stress on the body and nervous system.

What Does Chronic Stress Do to Your Body?

If you ask what is the single most important key to longevity, I would have to say it is avoiding worry, stress and tension. And if you didn't ask me, I'd still have to say it.
~George Burns

Stress affects every system of the body. Our bodies are not designed to handle chronic stress.

We need some time to recuperate after a period of stress, during which the parasympathetic nervous system takes over to restore homeostasis. Unfortunately, in our modern lifestyle, chronic stress is all too common. One of the harmful effects of chronic stress is subluxation.

Essentially, subluxation occurs when a spinal joint gets jarred out of a healthy position, either through trauma or unhealthy habits or a combination of the two. The affected tissues get squeezed and twisted, leading to injury, inflammation and nerve irritation.

This, in turn, disrupts the flow of information between your body and your brain and vice versa. This information is essential to keep you healthy and to heal your body. When it is disturbed, it affects your health. If this disruption of vital information continues long enough and is not corrected, it eventually results in symptoms. So, symptoms tend to show up at the end and not the beginning of the problem.

Nerves exit the spine through tiny holes, which also contain fatty tissue, blood vessels and lymph vessels. Any decrease in the hole size causes all of them to be compressed, but the nerves are the most sensitive. The signal through the nerve can be reduced by 10 per cent by 10 mm of pressure on a nerve, which is about the weight of a 5-cent coin!

Every time a vertebra misaligns, there is pressure on the spinal cord and nerve exiting the space between the spinal bones. This results in that body part receiving distorted signals from the innate intelligence centre in the brain. The reason why chiropractic care helps so many people with peripheral problems like muscle tension, muscle weakness, digestive problems and other issues is because it removes the interference in the communication network between those body parts and the brain.

Subluxation stress response

The main signs and symptoms of the subluxation stress response are:

- **Restricted motion:** Spinal joints get "stuck" and lose their normal range of motion.
- **Muscle tension:** Muscles surrounding the joint become tight to protect the joint from further damage.
- **Inflammation:** The body produces swelling around the abnormal joint to protect it from further damage.
- **Nerve pressure:** The abnormal movement, tight muscles, and swelling compress the spinal nerves. This interferes with the nerve signals communicating between your brain and body, leading to nerve damage and dysfunction.
- **Harmful effects:** If not corrected soon, this problem leads to degeneration of the spine and many other symptoms depending on the area affected.

The stress subluxation hypothesis states that vertebral subluxation constitutes a neurological stressor that activates the amygdala's stress response at a low level, chronically.

Four phases of spinal degeneration

What happens when your body can't deal with the subluxation?

Phase 1: In the first phase of subluxation degeneration, the spine's normal curvature is affected. The spine may not be damaged, but there may be a difference in the disc spacing. Usually, there is no pain. But without proper chiropractic care, the spine will continue to misalign, which leads to Phase Two of spinal degeneration.

Phase 2: In the second phase, along with misalignment, the normal curve of the spine is lost, and there is a narrowing of disc spaces. This may lead to backache, stiffness and limited range of motion. Again, chiropractic care may help to restore normal functioning. However, the damage to the discs and bones may be irreversible.

Phase 3: In the third phase, without proper care, there is spinal fusion. Degeneration of the spine worsens, which can cause permanent disc damage and an abnormal spinal curve. Chiropractic care in this phase can relieve symptoms and slow or stop the progression of spinal degeneration.

Phase 4: Both quality of life and longevity is reduced. The affected vertebrae become fused, which leads to permanent bone and nerve damage. The range of motion of the back becomes severely restricted.[14]

A simple chiropractic experiment

Get a rubber band and wind it several times around the base of your index finger until it is tight. The rubber band

---

[14] "Phases of Degeneration," Anchor Health Chiropractic, https://anchortohealth.com/degeneration/

does not cause any pain though that it has reduced the circulation to your finger. Initially, it won't affect your daily routine much.

Gradually, the lack of blood supply will cause problems in your finger due to cell damage. If you don't take off the rubber band, eventually, the finger will develop gangrene, and you may die of blood poisoning.

You can try various other options: ice pack, heat, massage, anti-inflammatory drugs or pain killers, magnets, acupressure, acupuncture, immobilisation, exercise, physiotherapy and so on. But only one thing will restore the blood supply to your finger and reverse the damage. And that is: remove the rubber band.

So, what is the best time to remove the rubber band from your finger? When your finger becomes numb? When it becomes gangrenous? After they amputate the gangrenous finger? Or when you are close to death? The answer is—**immediately**. Remove the rubber band as soon as you realise it is wrapped tightly around your finger.

Similarly, the best time to have your vertebral subluxations corrected is immediately!

Vertebral subluxations are misalignments of the bones in your spinal column. They compress nerve tissue and disturb the transmission of nerve impulses to their target cells, tissues and organs.

And just like the tight rubber band around your finger, vertebral subluxations may not cause any symptoms in the beginning. However, they are infinitely more harmful than a rubber band around your finger. They affect your body chemistry and your ability to adapt to stressors and heal naturally.

Chiropractors are the only healthcare providers who are trained to locate and correct subluxations. You may get a subluxation at any time and at any age. So, it's advisable to get your spine checked for vertebral subluxations regularly. It will improve your health and the quality of your life.

By the way, if you haven't already done so, remove the rubber band from your finger before going on to the next chapter. There we'll take a closer look at **subluxations**, the root cause of most health problems.

What is the Root Cause of Most Health Problems?

*X-rays will show misalignment that might cause
subluxation that causes nerve pressure.*
~Dr Clarence Selmer Gonstead

You may have heard of subluxation, but unless you've had personal experience with subluxation, you may not understand the damage it can cause.

Subluxation is a misalignment of the bones of the spinal column. It is definitely harmful to your health and should be corrected. Some of the common symptoms caused by subluxation are:

1. Backache or neck pain
This is the most common symptom of subluxation. Pain is felt either in the neck, in the back or both. Different people experience the pain differently. Some feel mild

discomfort, while others feel excruciating pain. If you have pain in the neck or back, it might be due to subluxation.

2. Stiffness and immobility
Subluxation causes pain that can make it difficult to move and perform ordinary tasks. The pain may discourage you from exercising, which can make the stiffness worse. If your back stiffness worsens, consult a chiropractor and get your spine checked and get the misalignment corrected.

3. Headaches
Spinal misalignments cause pressure and tension that may reach the base of the head and result in headaches. If you suffer from persistent headaches without any known cause, you need to check for a subluxation.

Poor posture types

1. Text neck ("tech neck")
Thanks to modern technology, we spend more and more time in front of our laptops and smartphones. Even everyday activities such as driving and brushing our teeth cause us to draw our heads forward and compress the small joints, discs and muscles that support our head.

The neck has an essential role in supporting the head and nervous system. It consists of seven bones called cervical vertebrae. They are separated by intervertebral discs, which act as shock absorbers and also provide nutrition. In addition, ligaments and muscles provide stability and mobility. This results in the neck being strong as well as flexible and mobile.

The neck has been designed to be positioned in a C shape. This position maintains its strength and mobility. However, we now spend a lot of time holding our heads forward and downwards at a 45-degree angle. This places a large amount of stress on our neck and shoulders.

When we constantly overload the neck by holding our head forward and down, it starts to damage its joints, discs and nerves. It also changes the normal C alignment of the neck. Once we lose this normal curvature, our spine is far more vulnerable to weakening and damage. The more we lose this normal shape, the more our joints, muscles, discs and even nerves are impacted and damaged.

Common symptoms of text neck include pain, stiffness, aching, numbness, sharp pain, shooting pain and even reduced mobility in both the neck and shoulders.

If text neck is ignored, symptoms will worsen with time and eventually lead to osteoarthritis and degenerative disc disease conditions.

The treatment of text neck first requires a proper diagnosis, including full physical testing, neurological testing and X-rays if indicated. Once its cause and stage are determined, an appropriate treatment plan can be designed.

While text neck is not easy to avoid in today's modern society, its long-term effects are not yet fully understood.

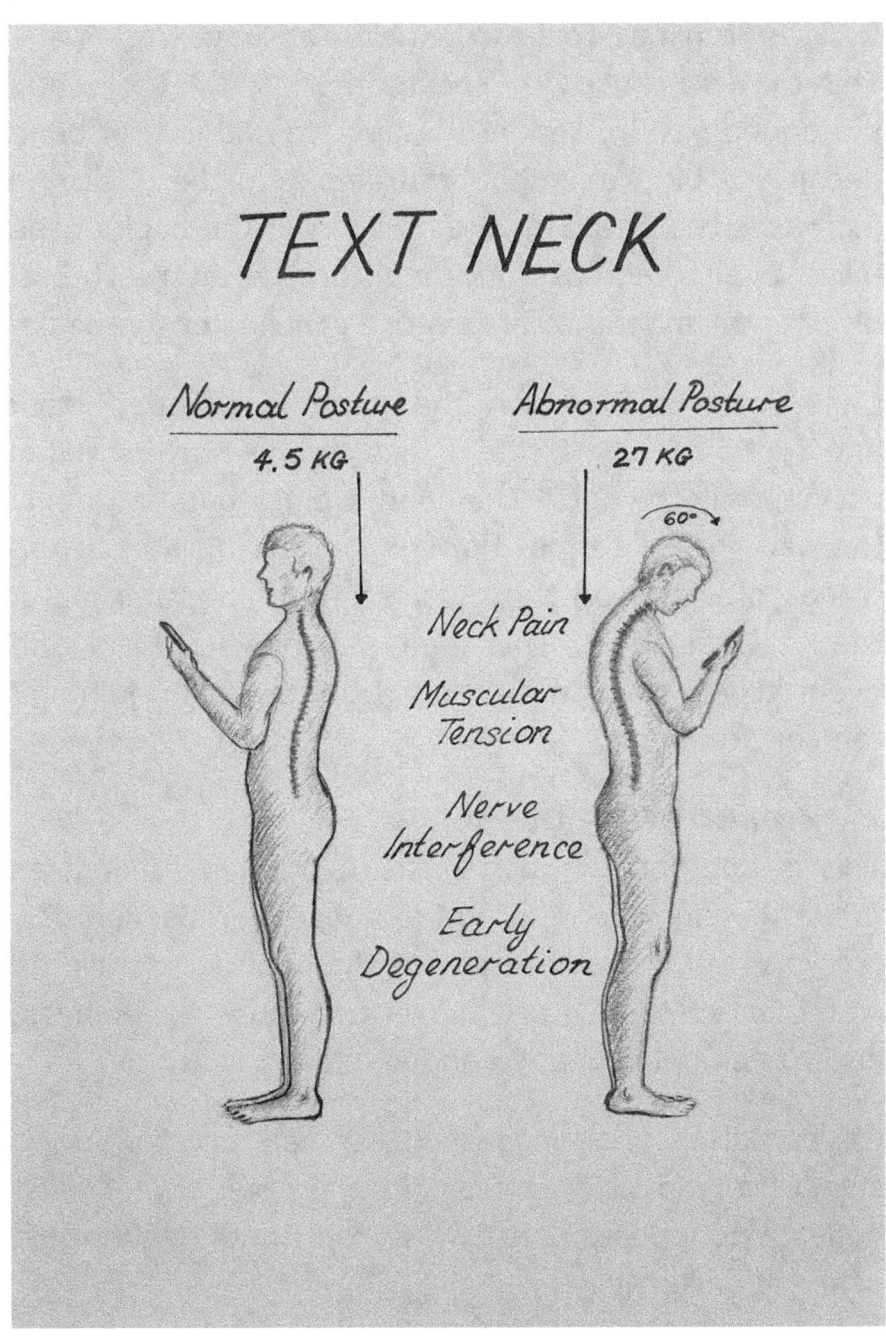

Diagram 3: text neck

2. Slouching or forward head posture

This may be caused by sports injuries, car accidents, prolonged sitting, sedentary lifestyle and loss of bone density. It blocks lymphatic drainage in the neck and increases the strain on the muscles in the back of the neck. It also increases the load on the intervertebral discs and can lead to premature arthritis of the neck.

Car accidents in which the head is whipped back and forward may suffer a loss of the normal spinal curvature in the neck. The head, weighing in at roughly the same as a tenpin bowling ball, is displaced and places pressure on the muscles, discs and nerves of the cervical spine. This leads to muscle strain and eventually to uneven wearing of the discs and joints of the cervical spine.

3. Forward tilt of the pelvis

This is another common posture problem. It causes forward weight bearing and increases lumbar lordosis (curvature). The abnormal weight bearing associated with this type of posture can lead to muscle weakness, lower back pain, sciatica and spinal arthritis.

Chiropractors analyse posture, spinal curvatures and spinal problems. They search for problems that exist beneath poor posture and which contribute to abnormal postural patterns.

For example, they look for changes in the stance, such as gait changes, tilting of the head and neck, height differences across the shoulders, levelling of the hips and pelvis, alignment of the knees and the outward turning of one or both feet.

In the next chapter, we'll take a closer look at the functioning of the nervous system, especially the sympathetic and parasympathetic systems.

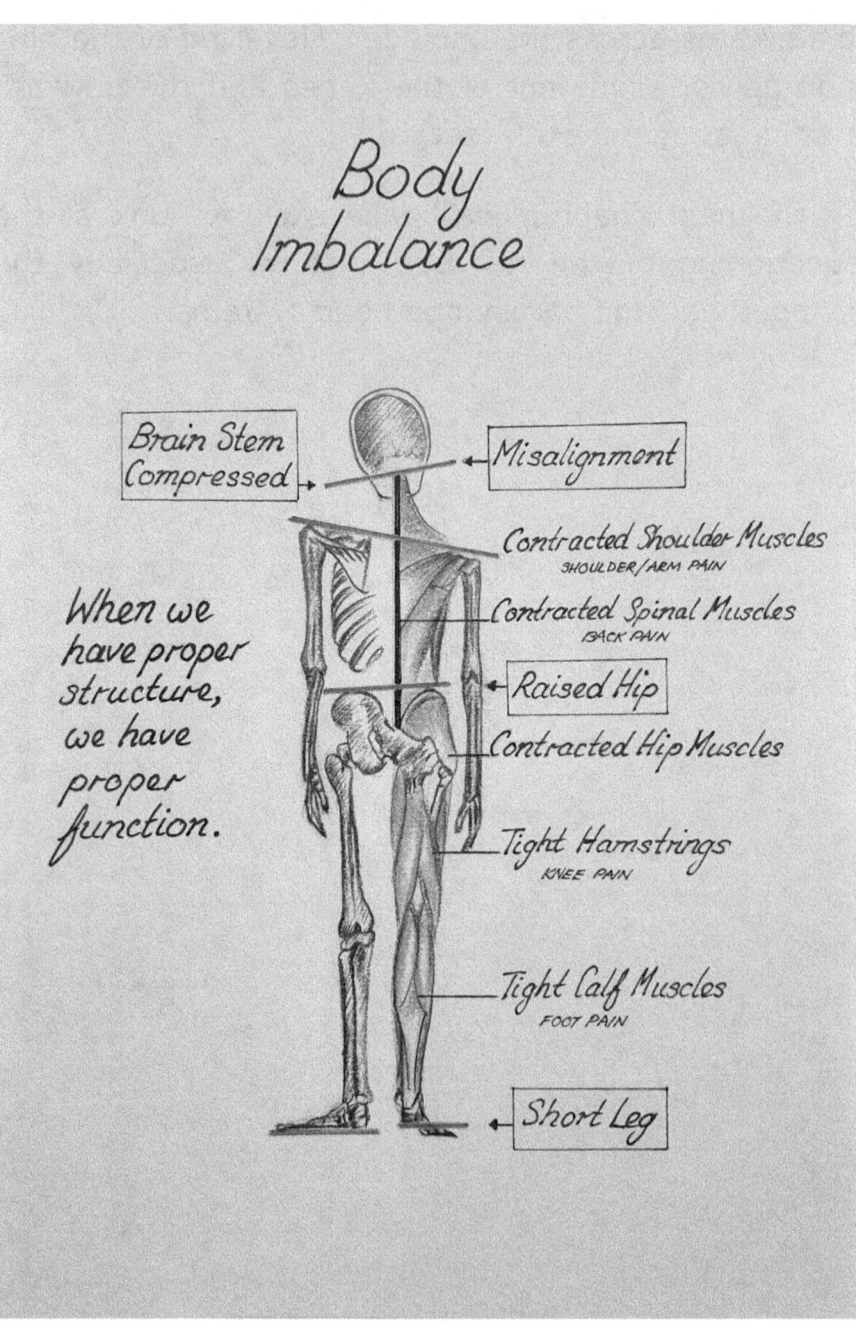

Diagram 4: body imbalance

How is Your Nervous System Functioning?

A universal lattice surrounds us that interacts with our sympathetic and parasympathetic nervous system.
~Laurence Galian

Sympathetic and parasympathetic systems

The sympathetic part of the central nervous system activates our "fight or flight" mode in response to stress. When the sympathetic system is activated, it stimulates the release of the hormone epinephrine (also known as adrenaline) into the bloodstream.

Epinephrine brings about the following physiological changes:

- Our heart beats faster and pumps more blood to the muscles, heart and other vital organs. So, our heart rate and blood pressure increase.

- Small airways in our lungs open wider, and we start to breathe more rapidly so that we can take in more oxygen with every breath. The extra oxygen is sent to the brain and makes us more alert.
- Our blood sugar and fats increase to supply more energy to all parts of the body, especially to the muscles.
- Our vision, hearing and other senses become razor-sharp.

The sympathetic stimulation puts our body into survival mode (the flight or fight response). Now, this response is sometimes necessary. However, an excessive sympathetic response is harmful and affects our focus. Prolonged sympathetic stimulation can lead to fatigue, anxiety and sleep disturbances, etc.[15]

The parasympathetic system has the opposite response: it is responsible for resting and digesting, it slows the body down and calms it so that it can repair itself and heal from stress, sickness or injury. So, we can say that the parasympathetic response is essential for good health and recovery.

Both the sympathetic and parasympathetic systems are vital for health, but they affect us in different ways. An imbalance between these two systems can lead

---

[15] "Understanding the stress response," Harvard Health Publishing, last updated 6 July 2020, https://www.health.harvard.edu/staying-healthy/understanding-the-stress-response.

to health problems. So, we need to ensure a balance between these two systems.

Restore balance through chiropractic care

Chiropractic care is so much more than addressing and improving musculoskeletal health such as backache and neuropathy. Chiropractic care does much more. It improves the health of the entire nervous system, that is, both the sympathetic and parasympathetic systems.

It's difficult to separate chiropractic from stress because these stressors cause subluxation. However, chiropractors not only understand how stress impacts the movements of the spine—they are trained to see the broader picture and how stress impacts the whole system.

A study carried out by researchers at the Sherman College of Straight Chiropractic suggests that cervical adjustments may result in parasympathetic responses, and thoracic adjustments may result in sympathetic responses. Hence, this study demonstrates the relationship of responses to the segments adjusted.[16]

Chiropractic care may correct stresses on the nerves that lead to an imbalance of the nervous system. Gentle spinal adjustments can reduce and remove nerve

---

[16] A Welch and R Boone, "Sympathetic and Parasympathetic Responses to Specific Diversified Adjustments to Chiropractic Vertebral Subluxations of the Cervical And Thoracic Spine," *Journal of Chiropractic Medicine* 7, no. 3 (2008): 86–93, https://doi.org/10.1016/j.jcm.2008.04.001.

compression that activates the sympathetic system. Regular chiropractic brings the body back into balance so it can begin to heal itself.

Chiropractic care helps keep the central nervous system in balance, reduces dysfunction, and improves overall health. Unfortunately, the most common way that these signals are disrupted is through subluxations. Next, let's see how to correct these disruptions within our nervous system.

How to Correct Problems with Your Nervous System?

Chiropractic is designed not only to make you instantly feel better, but also to make you instantly heal better.
~Unknown

Chiropractic care is the best way to correct a subluxation of the spine. Chiropractors use spinal manipulation to adjust the vertebrae of the spine back into their proper places. They eliminate the symptoms caused by subluxation; better still, they bring about other health benefits.

Most people don't understand the benefits and safety of chiropractic. They seek chiropractic only when they are in pain and after they have tried all other available treatment options, as if the chiropractor is a panel beater that needs to put them back together, but the wiser approach is to think of your chiropractor as a

Formula-1 technician that provides fine tuning so that you can perform at your best.

The safety pin cycle is a simple communication tool to illustrate the remarkable power of your nervous system and the equally significant healing power of a chiropractic adjustment.

Every safety pin has four parts, each of which represents an aspect of the chiropractic model of health:

- The left side represents nerve impulses from the brain to the body.
- The right side represents nerve impulses returning to the brain from the body.
- The clasp represents the brain.
- The spring represents the body.

The clasped safety pin represents uninterrupted nerve communication between the brain and body in both directions, essential for good health and wellbeing.

The unclasped safety pin represents ill health caused by impaired nerve connection between the brain and the body. This can be on the side from the brain to the body or to the brain from the body. This is called vertebral subluxation. Even the slightest spinal misalignment can have neurological effects.

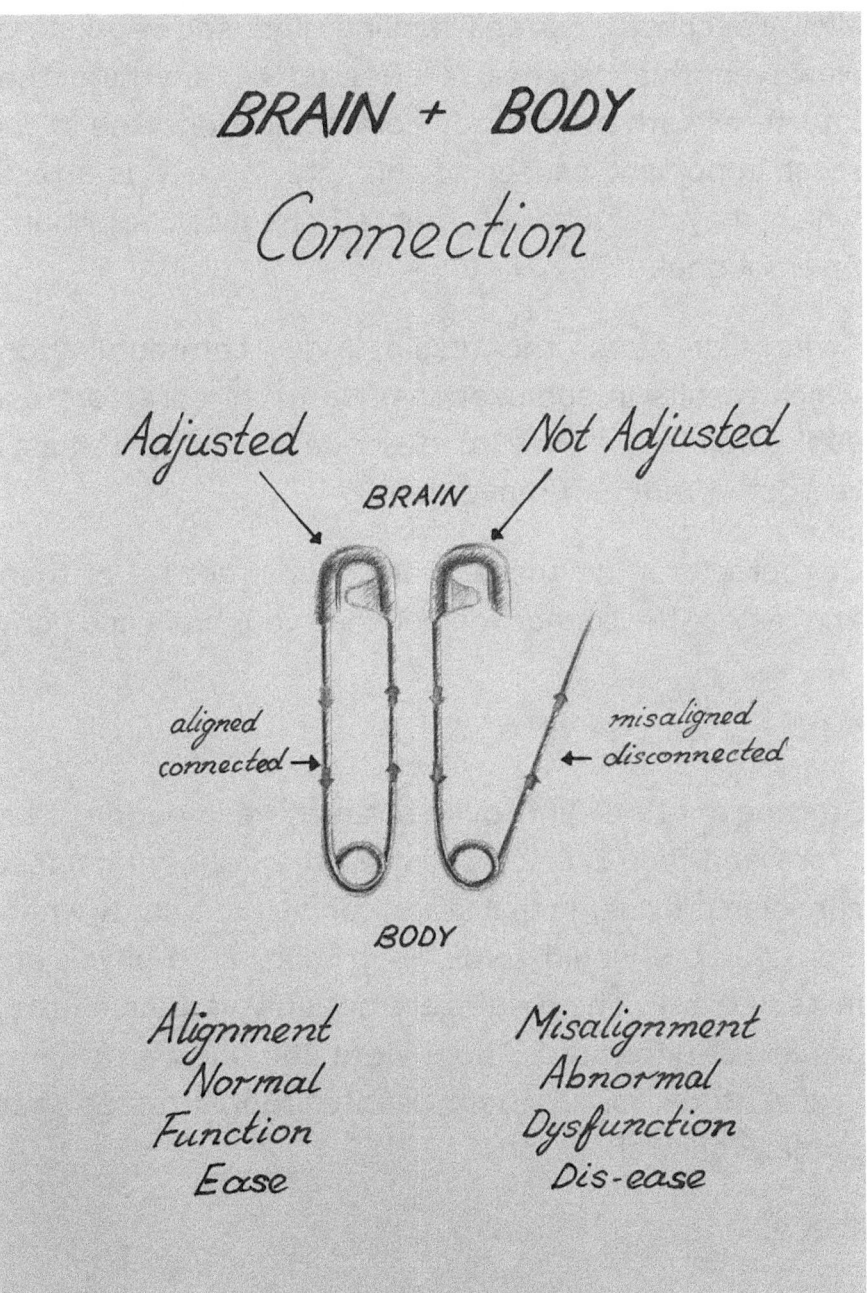

Diagram 5: The Safety Pin Cycle

We are constantly self-healing and self-regulating. However, this process is affected by anything that interferes with brain–body communication. One of the most important causes of this interference is stress, which may be physical, mental, chemical, nutritional or emotional.

Stress disrupts the brain–body communication, which results in subluxations. Many chiropractors use subluxation as a way to describe a joint that has a restricted range of movement.

Chiropractors find these subluxations, get rid of them and restore the connection between your brain and body.

Blue Cross Shield study

Starting in 1999 and over a seven-year period, Blue Cross and Blue Shield of Illinois, the largest managed care plan provider in that state, conducted a study where chiropractors would serve as primary care physicians in its network. The results are not only verifiable—they are as yet unrefuted. There were 700,000 participants in this study, all of whom used chiropractors as their primary care physicians.

The results of this study were:

- Hospitalisation was reduced by approximately 60%
- Outpatient surgery and procedures were reduced by approximately 85%

- Pharmaceutical (drug) use was reduced by approximately 56%
- Zero C-section births were delivered (compared to a 22% average outside this program).

The results of his study surprised even the researchers who conducted it: "I have always believed that the over-utilisation of pharmaceuticals and surgery, and the under-utilisation of more natural healing techniques, like chiropractic, have been the cause of great suffering. Yet, I had no idea that magnitude of both clinical improvements and cost-effectiveness would approach 50% in both cases", Keith Pendleton, "DCs and Diagnosis"[17] [18]

Finally, let's examine when the best time is to start taking care of your health. There is an ancient Chinese saying that applies to your health, "The best time to plant a tree is twenty years ago. The next best time is now."

---

[17] RL Sarnat & Winterstein, "Clinical and Cost Outcomes of an Integrative Medicine IPA, *Journal of Manipulative Physiological Therapies* 27, no. 5 (June 2004): 336–47, http://doi.org/10.1016/j.jmpt.2004.04.007.

[18] RL Sarnat, J Winterstein & JA Cambron, "Clinical Utilization and Cost Outcomes from an Integrative Medicine Independent Physician Association: An Additional 3-Year Update, *Journal of Manipulative Physiological Therapies* 30 no. 4 (May 2007): 263–9, https://doi.org/10.1016/j.jmpt.2007.03.004.

When is the Best Time to Take Care of Your Health?

The doctor of the future will give no medicine, but will instruct his patients in the care of the human frame, in diet, and in the cause and prevention of disease.
~Thomas Edison

You have probably heard the old Dutch saying: "Prevention is better than cure". It's absolutely true. Prevention is indeed the best medicine. You may think that prevention of disease means a healthy diet, regular exercise, good sleep, adequate hydration and proper stress management. And you would be quite right.

However, if you really want to take your health to the next level, consider these reasons why chiropractic care might be the best way to prevent illness and promote health.

1. Chiropractic may reduce present pain and help prevent future pain

Pain is inevitable, but suffering is not. As we age, our bodies tend to become stiff and sore. Chiropractors correct spinal misalignments that are associated with pain. Though they may be unable to eliminate all pain completely, they *can* minimise current pain all the while reducing the risk of future pain associated with mechanical joint dysfunction.

2. Chiropractic care improves spine health and overall wellbeing

The healthier the spine, the healthier the body. By healing and boosting the spine's health, chiropractic care produces a sense of wellbeing and improves all aspects of life.

3. Chiropractic improves your immunity and capacity to heal

The best way to be healthy is to enhance your body's natural immune system. The central nervous system relays important information to other systems, including the immune system, to keep them working properly. By taking care of the spine with chiropractic care, you're boosting the Central Nervous System as well as the immune system and other systems that depend on it.

Truly, an ounce of prevention is better than a tonne of treatment, and the "journey of a thousand miles begins with a single step". So, the sooner you consult your chiropractor, the sooner you can take the first step to improve your health and quality of life.

Universal Truths

*The secret of good health lies in successful
adjustment to changing stresses on the body.
~Harry J. Johnson*

How will you feel if your car breaks down by the side of the road while you are on your way to a really important appointment? You will probably feel stress, frustration, distress and a regret too deep for words.

You ignored the fact that your car was giving you distress signals. You were too preoccupied and too busy to call a mechanic. Now you are paying the price for this wilful neglect: unnecessary misery, profound inconvenience and expensive repairs.

You fear your car may never be the same again—even after it is repaired. You should have called the mechanic before the problem snowballed.

There is a close relationship between your car and your body. How you care for each very much affects how they operate.

Similar to your car, your body is breaking down from wear and tear and neglect. You have two options:

1. You can continue to neglect your body until it breaks down. This option is as short-term as it is short-sighted. Plus, unlike cars, there are no spare parts for your body.
2. Check for early signs of ill health and act immediately to make small lifestyle changes that can improve your health drastically. Consult a chiropractor for adjustments, physical therapy and the like so that your body stays fine-tuned to perform at its best. Then, should you fall ill or become injured, you still have the capacity to heal fully and recover quickly.

Scheduled visits to your chiropractor

Your car needs to be serviced regularly by a skilled mechanic so that the different oils, for example, can be changed and all parts checked to ensure performance and prevent any future problems.

Similarly, you need to visit your chiropractor for care based on assessing your current health and preventing future health problems. If your current health care provider cannot provide a satisfactory solution, seek out a second opinion.

A nutritious and balanced diet

If you don't add fuel to the car, it will stop running. Also, you must use high-quality fuel. Low-quality fuel will affect the performance of your car and cause the motor to run rough, increase speed slowly and probably emit toxic fumes. Long-term use of low-quality fuel may irreversibly damage the motor.

Similarly, a healthy diet is vital for your health. Poor quality nutrients such as sugary and deep-fried foods may be cheap, convenient and enjoyable, but they will definitely damage your health and physical fitness. Over time, they can lead to dangerous disorders like obesity, diabetes, high blood pressure, heart disease and stroke.

Respect the reality of your ageing body

However, don't go to the other extreme and become overcautious. Many seniors restrict themselves to a short stroll and are wary of trying different activities. Make sure you respond wisely to the changing needs and desires of your body. Do regular resistance training to prevent decreasing muscle mass. Practise balancing activities to minimise the chances of a fall. Join a yoga class to reduce body stiffness and improve the range of motion of your joints.

Everything breaks down with time. This is true of both your car and your body. However, if you plan properly and make wise and positive actions under the guidance of a skilled professional, you can enjoy a long and carefree life.[19]

---

[19] G Conian, "Your body, the motor vehicle, and the law of entropy," Living Now, last modified 17 September 2018, https://livingnow.com.au/body-motor-vehicle-law-entropy/.

Fibs, Tales and Lies

*The power that made the body heals the
body. It happens no other way.*
~B. J. Palmer

Some common misconceptions about chiropractic are:

Myth #1: Chiropractors are not real doctors

Chiropractors in Australia receive their title of "Dr" through national registration with their professional body. This is similar to other healthcare professionals. In addition, chiropractors are professionals subject to the same testing procedures, licensing and monitoring by national peer-reviewed boards, similar to medical doctors.

Doctors of chiropractic receive their registration through the Australian Health Practitioner Regulation Agency. This body also registers other mainstream healthcare providers such as GPs, dentists, physiotherapists, psychologists and podiatrists.

The Department of Veterans' Affairs, Medicare and Workers' Compensation programs cover chiropractic care, and medical (sick-leave) certificates signed by chiropractors are accepted everywhere.

Chiropractors undergo five years of university-based training and education. They will have delivered hundreds of adjustments in their final year of studies under the supervision of registered chiropractic doctors before graduating. Their studies are similar to those of medical schools; their rigorous curricula covers anatomy, physiology, cell biology, pathophysiology, chemistry, biochemistry, immunology, physical examination, diagnostic skills, physical therapies and rehabilitation.

As primary health practitioners, chiropractors are sometimes the first healthcare contact for a patient and are trained to identify situations where the patient may need medical or other care.

Chiropractors are licensed to practise as health care providers in many countries worldwide, including the USA, UK, Canada, Switzerland, Australia and New Zealand.

The most significant difference between chiropractors and medical doctors is their preferred method of caring for people rather than their level of education. On the other hand, medical doctors are trained in the practice of medicine and surgery. So they can be beneficial in medical and surgical conditions such as infections, appendicitis, fractures, strokes, cancers, etc.

However, if you have restricted joint movement, especially in your spine or soft tissue damage causing pain, it cannot be fixed by chemicals. At the most, painkillers may provide temporary relief, but they cannot cure the underlying cause.

Physical problems such as these need a physical solution. Chiropractors help the body heal by providing physical solutions for physical conditions (e.g., muscle spasms and backache) and headaches that consist of adjustments, exercises, physical therapy, stretches, etc.[20]

Myth #2: Medical doctors don't like chiropractors

Historically, vocal opponents of chiropractic have been shown to have had hidden agendas.

Morris Fishbein led the American Medical Association (AMA)'s opposition to chiropractic in the 1940s. Fishbein presented chiropractors as mercenary members of an unscientific cult. He called them "rabid dogs."

---

[20] "Chiropractic Myths" Dr Princetta, https://drprincetta.com/chiro-myths/.

The conventional medical establishment conspired to defame and destroy the chiropractic profession. Fast forward to the 1980s, and a landmark lawsuit in the Supreme Court of Illinois found the AMA guilty of conspiracy, ordering them to pay restitution to the chiropractic profession.[21]

Closer to home, a report commissioned by the New Zealand Government in 1978 developed into the most comprehensive and detailed independent examination of chiropractic ever undertaken in any country at that time. The focus of the investigation was to consider whether health and accident benefits should be made available for chiropractic services.

When this report was commissioned, it was believed only a month or two, at most, would be needed to resolve the issues. However, it took nearly two years, generating over 3,600 pages of testimony under oath from numerous witnesses and thousands of pages of document submissions from organisations and private parties across the globe.

Much of the so-called evidence by self-appointed consumer rights advocates and very vocal medical experts was found to be "fraudulent" or "pure propaganda", and the expert statements were labelled "highly unreliable" by the Royal Commission.

---

[21] "U.S. Judge Finds Medical Group Conspired Against Chiropractors," *New York Times*, 29 August 1987, https://www.nytimes.com/1987/08/29/us/us-judge-finds-medical-group-conspired-against-chiropractors.html.

The investigators also travelled to Canada, the US, the UK and Australia to quest for information. Finally, the lengthy report was presented in September 1979, with favourable findings about chiropractic and manipulation. Similar results were later published in the Rand Study, the Meade Report, the British Medical Journal, the Magna Report, the ACHPR Report on back pain and numerous subsequent research journal studies.

In the 40-plus years since then, the opinion of many medical doctors about chiropractic has changed.

Several major studies have confirmed the efficacy of chiropractic in helping people with a wide range of conditions. Most medical doctors understand much better what chiropractors actually do.

Also, many people have informed their medical doctors about the benefits they have experienced with chiropractic care. Many hospitals in the US now have chiropractors on staff, and some chiropractic offices have medical doctors on staff. Chiropractic students in Australia are occasionally taught by academic staff with medical or dual qualification.

The end result is that medical doctors and chiropractors are much more likely to team up and collaborate in cases where medical and chiropractic care complement each other.

Myth #3: You have to go to a chiropractor for the rest of your life

Going to a chiropractor is much like eating healthy food, attending a yoga class or going to the dentist. You do it because you want to enjoy the benefits. Similarly, you go to your chiropractor's office because you want to maintain your good health.

For example, doctors tell their patients that an annual check-up at the clinic will help detect illnesses like high blood pressure, diabetes and even early-stage cancer. Similarly, dentists tell their patients that an annual dental check-up will help take care of their teeth more effectively. In the same way, regular visits to your chiropractor will maintain the health of your neuromusculoskeletal and nervous system.

Your spine undergoes normal wear and tear even during your routine daily activities. But, more importantly, the stress we experience because of the increasing complexity in our lives often manifests as pain in our bodies. We see this in practice each and every day, with highly stressed people often presenting with headaches, neck and/or back pain.

Regular chiropractic care helps you move with more freedom, manage stress better, and maintain good health throughout your life. So you can improve your health even with short-term chiropractic care. However, if you choose to make chiropractic care a part of your wellness lifestyle, you will enjoy abundant and lasting benefits. In this respect, chiropractic care is like compound interest; the longer the period, the more exponential the gains.

Myth #4: Cracking bones are scraping together

During a back adjustment, you may hear a cracking or popping noise when your back undergoes gentle stretching of the spinal facet joints. This popping sound is caused by small pockets of air, which are present in the fluid surroundings of these joints. When the joints are stretched during a chiropractic adjustment, the pockets of air *pop*, which creates that cracking sound. So, don't be worried about the popping sounds you hear during a spinal adjustment.[22]

Myth #5: Chiropractic care is dangerous

One of the safest types of health care in the world is chiropractic care. According to the WHO, when employed skilfully and appropriately, chiropractic care is safe and effective for preventing and managing a number of health problems.[23]

---

[22] S Haldeman, *Principles and Practice of Chiropractic*, (York, PA: McGraw-Hill, 2005).

[23] "WHO guidelines on basic training and safety in chiropractic," World Health Organization, 2005, https://www.who.int/medicines/areas/traditional/Chiro-Guidelines.pdf.

You only need to compare the malpractice premiums paid by chiropractors to those paid by medical doctors. Doctors of Chiropractic pay only about 1/20th of the amount paid by medical doctors in malpractice premiums.

Medical errors are the third leading cause of death in the US[24]. Yet, on the other hand, out of the millions of people receiving chiropractic adjustments each year, very few will even make a complaint.[25]

So, these myths about chiropractic care are completely untrue. In fact, chiropractic care provides natural, pain-free healing for optimum health and quality of life.

---

[24] B Starfield, "Is US Health Really the Best in the World? JAMA 284 no. 4 (2000): 483–485, https://doi.org/10.1001/jama.284.4.483.

[25] "Busted! Don't Believe These Chiropractic Care Myths!" last updated 24 October 2017, https://www.torontochiropracticservices.com/blogs/blog/160142-busted--don-t-believe-these-chiropractic-care-myths#.YEtXPZvhVLM.

A New Beginning ...

> **Health is the new wealth.**
> We will still define success by how nice our house is or the zip code we live in. But going forward, health is going to become increasingly synonymous with social status. Health will be a currency of its own. You cannot necessarily buy health, but you will know how to earn it, and you earn it every day of your life.
> ~Henry Loubet, CEO, Bohemia Health

Congratulations on finishing the book! Whether you read every chapter or read the topics of interest to you (or just skimmed your way to this page), you are taking action.

Now that you have read my book and learned the 10 questions to unlock your abundant health, I invite you to take the next step.

Attend a free, no-obligation workshop and learn how to restore your inner awesomeness with chiropractic.

Simply register at mychiro.com.au/workshop or scan the image below:

And check out my website: https://www.mychiro.com.au/

All the best for your journey towards a vibrant and healthy life.

Gratefully,

Steve

Dr Steven Lockstone
B.App.Sc.(Clin.Sc.)/B.C.Sc. RMIT
Chiropractor | Wellness Influencer | Speaker

Connect with me: mychiro.com.au/drsteve

References

Alford, H. "The Tyranny of Constant Contact." *New York Times*. Last modified 17 May 2015. https://www.nytimes.com/2015/05/17/style/the-tyranny-of-constant-contact.html.

Anchor Health Chiropractic 2016. "Phases of Degeneration." https://anchortohealth.com/degeneration/.

Australian Institute of Health and Welfare. "Deaths in Australia." Last modified 7 August 2020. https://www.aihw.gov.au/reports/life-expectancy-death/deaths/data.

Australian Institute of Health and Welfare. "Accidental drug overdose deaths up almost 40 per cent in a decade." Last modified 27 August 2019. https://www.abc.net.au/news/health/2019-08-27/accidental-drug-overdoses-forecast-to-reach-record-high/11450764.

Australian Spinal Research Foundation. "The Stress Series: Part 1 – Stress Physiology – A Central Theme in Chiropractic? https://spinalresearch.com.au/

the-stress-series-part-1-stress-physiology-a-central-theme-in-chiropractic/.

Conian, G. "Your body, the motor vehicle, and the law of entropy." Living Now. Last modified 17 September 2018. https://livingnow.com.au/body-motor-vehicle-law-entropy/.

Franki, R. "Comorbidities the rule in New York's COVID-19 deaths." The Hospitalist. 2020. https://www.the-hospitalist.org/hospitalist/article/220457/coronavirus-updates/comorbidities-rule-new-yorks-covid-19-deaths.

Garg S, L Kim, M Whitaker, A O'Halloran and C Cummings et al. "Hospitalization rates and characteristics of patients hospitalized with laboratory-confirmed coronavirus disease 2019 — COVID-NET, 14 states, March 1–30, 2020." *MMWR Morbidity & Mortality Weekly Report* 69 (2020): 458–464. http://dx.doi.org/10.15585/mmwr.mm6915e3.

Haldeman, S. *Principles and Practice of Chiropractic*. York, PA: McGraw-Hill, 2005.

Harvard Health Publishing. "Understanding the stress response." Last updated 6 July 2020. https://www.health.harvard.edu/staying-healthy/understanding-the-stress-response.

New York Times. "U.S. Judge Finds Medical Group Conspired Against Chiropractors." 9 August 1987.

https://www.nytimes.com/1987/08/29/us/us-judge-finds-medical-group-conspired-against-chiropractors.html.

Paudel, SS. "A Meta-Analysis of 2019 Novel Coronavirus Patient Clinical Characteristics and Comorbidities." *Research Square* (2020). http://doi.org/10.21203/rs.3.rs-21831/v1.

Princetta, P. "Chiropractic Myths". Dr Princetta. https://drprincetta.com/chiro-myths/.

Sanyaolu, A., C Okorie, A Marinkovic, R Patidar, K Younis, P Desai, Z Hosein, I Padda, J Mangat and M Altaf. Comorbidity and its Impact on Patients with COVID-19. *SN Comprehensive Clinical Medicine*. (2020): 1–8. Advance online publication. https://doi.org/10.1007/s42399-020-00363-4

The Skill Collective. "5 reasons why modern life causes stress (and what to do about it)." Last updated 29 May 2017. https://theskillcollective.com/blog/modern-life-causes-stress.

Toronto Chiropractic Servicea. "Busted! Don't Believe These Chiropractic Care Myths!". 24 October 2017. https://www.torontochiropracticservices.com/blogs/blog/160142-busted--don-t-believe-these-chiropractic-care-myths#.YEtXPZvhVLM.

Sarnat RL and J Winterstein. "Clinical and Cost Outcomes of an Integrative Medicine IPA, *Journal of Manipulative*

Physiological Therapies 27, no. 5 (June 2004): 336–47. http://doi.org/10.1016/j.jmpt.2004.04.007.

Sarnat RL, J Winterstein and JA Cambron. "Clinical Utilization and Cost Outcomes from an Integrative Medicine Independent Physician Association: An Additional 3-Year Update." *Journal of Manipulative Physiological Therapies* 30, no. 4 (May 2007): 263–9. https://doi.org/10.1016/j.jmpt.2007.03.004.

Starfield B. "Is US Health Really the Best in the World? JAMA 284 no. 4 (2000): 483–485. https://doi.org/10.1001/jama.284.4.483.

Welch, A and R Boone. "Sympathetic and Parasympathetic Responses to Specific Diversified Adjustments to Chiropractic Vertebral Subluxations of the Cervical and Thoracic Spine." *Journal of Chiropractic Medicine* 7, no. 3 (2008): 86–93. https://doi.org/10.1016/j.jcm.2008.04.001.

World Health Organization. "Constitution." https://www.who.int/about/who-we-are/constitution

World Health Organization. "WHO guidelines on basic training and safety in chiropractic." 2005. https://www.who.int/medicines/areas/traditional/Chiro-Guidelines.pdf.